Jesus

Counsel

The Perfect Cocktail – Prayer, Counseling and Sometimes Medication.

By

Queen E. Lacey

Author of Sexually Driven

Published by Hemingway Publisher
ISBN: [XXXXXXXXXXXX]
Printed in United States of America

Dedication

*To all those that didn't judge me but
wanted the best for me.
Thank you so very much!*

About the Author

~

Author Queen Esther Lacey began her early years in the chilly region of White Plains, New York, prior to relocating to sunny Arizona in December 2001, where she now enjoys hot summers in the new land of promise. Of the fruit of her womb yields one son and one daughter who has yielded her two grandchildren. Battling through childhood depression, Queen Esther wrote through her plight after becoming inspired by a teacher who noted the gift of writing and gifted her with a book by author Langston Hughes. Throughout her journey of life, writing was always a part of what Queen Esther considers her "private life" until becoming the published author of her first work in 2009: "It's Not About Religion, God Wants a Relationship. God's Love is Unconditional," a thoughtful depiction of personal experiences and inspirations written in poetic form. Queen Esther has since authored and published eight books to date. Queen Esther is one who deeply cares for the hurting and is passionate about using her gift of writing to reach multitudes of women and minister healing and encouragement to all who are seeking to find hope in whatever situation they find themselves.

PEbyQueen@yahoo.com

Table of Contents

~

Introduction

My last publication was titled Injured and Scarred but Not Broken. The main thing I was trying to say with that was I had been through a lot of things in life, but it didn't leave me damaged.

When my mother passed away, it uncovered my fear of dying to an overwhelming level, but because of the last title, I couldn't share my struggle because I felt like that would make me a liar and that I'm not damaged or broken.

Yes, I'm saved, so I knew I could not take my life and not escape hell's fire. Yet still, I feared every day that one day the darkness would overtake me.

Was I a liar? Was I broken? Was I damaged goods? Maybe not broken, but not completely whole. We take medication for everything that ails us, so why is there such a stigma connected to something to balance the chemicals in the brain? Despite the stigma, today, I reached out for help. Am I still saved? Yes! I think about the scripture in Jerimiah 18. The vessel being marred but still in the hands of the potter (God's hand).

Having faith in a situation is good. However, faith without works is dead. Works can come in the form of medication and/or counseling. You can consult experts and doctors to gain knowledge about mental illness, I just want to share my testimony of how Jesus & Counsel (and sometimes medication) can be a winning combination.

BE ENCOURAGED EVERY DAY!!!

-Queen Esther Lacey

Chapter One

The Doctor's Diagnosis for Queen

~~~

Mental Illness:

Variants or mental disorders or, less commonly, mental diseases are any of a broad range of medical conditions (such as major depression, schizophrenia, obsessive-compulsive disorder, or panic disorder) that are marked primarily by sufficient disorganization of personality, mind, or emotions to impair normal psychological functioning and cause marked distress or disability and that are typically associated with a disruption in normal thinking, feeling, mood, behavior, interpersonal interactions, or daily functioning.

With the doctor diagnosing mental illness, it was felt group therapy and medication would be the answer to the question of what is going on with this child. My group therapy was about 4 or 5 children. We would meet at the hospital in what felt like a classroom. If I remember correctly, sometimes, we would sit in a circle and go around the room and talk about things. At the end of the session, we would have a snack. The therapy came more in-depth as I got older. I was seeing the therapist one on one in their office. Hospitalize three times because of depression and not wanting to live.

As I got older, more and more labels were added.

- Bipolar (Manic Depression)
- PTSD
- Social Anxiety Disorder
- ADD
- Basic Health Issues:
- High blood pressure
- Enlarged Heart
- Diabetic
- Thyroid
- High Cholesterol
- Kidney Disease

- Anemic

- Arthritis (Needing Knee Replacement)

*Note – I mention trigger throughout the pages – It means what sets me off and what causes me to explode or withdraw.

As a little black girl that was having a hard time dealing with life. Acting out and just misbehaving. The school system wants to label it as slow or special ED. Somehow I was seen by a therapist, and it was determined I had a chemical imbalance in my brain and would need group therapy and medication. I guess when you are a child, it is better to handle it as a group, and as I got older, it was through individual sessions.

Some think if you are depressed, you can just turn and be happy. But when there is a chemical imbalance, it takes medication to level that individual out. I don't know if medicating was easier, but I know I went through several dosages of different medications until they got it right. Sometimes it takes hospitalization as it did with me. I'll talk about that later.

Chapter Two

Queen and Bipolar (Manic Depression)

~

Bipolar Disorder (Manic Depression):

A mental illness in which a person experiences periods of strong excitement and happiness followed by periods of sadness and depression.

Court Experience:

The first time I must have been about 19 or 20, and CPS (Child Protective Services) took me to court. Apparently, someone reported me, stating I wasn't a good parent. There was a young representative that came to see me at my place of business and asked me a bunch of questions. I don't like answering those questions. She said you are young and don't want to be a parent. I shut down. I showed up to court and was so upset because the judge was beginning the same with the questions in a very degrading way. He would spell it out like I was stupid when he said do you understand?

That triggered my shutdown. Looking back now, maybe if I had been able to answer differently, I might not have lost custody. Once I go into depressed mode, I am not able to pull myself out.

Another time I was planning to move to AZ, one of my children said they wanted to come back home, and I told the father I needed the birth certificate to get the child enrolled in school. The next thing I knew, I was back in court. The agent for the child was asking me questions that triggered me. I went into a deep depression and couldn't shake it. The judge said the child was to be removed from the home immediately. I was in a state of shock. So, I didn't have custody of my children from elementary school. I am still trying to have a healthy relationship with them. It's not easy because I feel like I must watch what I say not to upset them. Do I have to pay the price for being a horrible mother for the rest of my life?

One day I would love to hear my children say they love me and celebrate me on birthdays, Mother's Day, and holidays. To meet up and go on trips would be awesome. But they live such different lives. I can't blame them; I just hope and dream.

Hospital Experience:

There were several times my actions landed me a shared room in the local hospital mental health ward. There was such a dark cloud over my life. I always used to write, not realizing it was a gift because my writing was so dark and depressing. I was just getting my feelings out.

I would go to a session with my doctor, and the doctor would feel I was a danger to myself and/or others.

There were times when I would cut myself. There were times I would save up my medication and plan to take it at once to end it all. There was a time I took the wrong drug that was laced with something that was detrimental to me.

I remember I found myself on a bridge during one of my night walks (I would walk the streets at night when I couldn't sleep). I was standing there thinking about jumping. Now, I'm afraid of bridges, and I was there like frozen. It must have been the Lord or just a coincidence that someone came by and ministered to me not to proceed.

Outside of the time with drugs, I would go through a therapy session, and they would suggest I be hospitalized. Right from the start, it was a humble experience. All my life, I have looked at it in a negative way. However, now, I can see how people were looking out for my safety. I have been hospitalized three times. It was like a prison to me. You are body searched and must change into simple clothes so that you can't hurt yourself. And you are watched around the clock. Yes, a prison.

When I ate, I had to sit at the nursing station for a length of time so that my food would digest long enough that I wouldn't bring it up. It was almost at the point that I was doing it so much I could will myself to throw up. I didn't have to stick my fingers down my throat.

It was explained having an eating disorder was a way of wanting to harm oneself as well. Having your freedom taken from you is never fun. I was always being watched. But again, it was for my safety. While in the hospital, I was put on SSI, so when I left the hospital, I didn't return to work and was treated as an outpatient.

Relationship Experience:

I can't really explain, but my thoughts about love were so warped. There would be days that I would feel so good I couldn't sit still. I didn't understand all my triggers. Then after I performed acts of giving my body to any random person, I would hit the very lows of depression.

The only way I can explain to you my struggle with sex is to share different episodes or adventures. I'll leave it up to you how you want to describe it. Just to give you a little understanding, sex is not a pleasurable loving experience for me; each experience brought a darker hate for it and for myself. In my mind, I wanted to be loved and feel like I was worth something, but more and more, I realized I was only good for one thing in life, and no one was going to love me.

As a child, we would go over different family members' homes, and sometimes I was left alone with cousins who would touch me in ways no child should be touched: both male and female. I never thought about it before, but they must have been touched too to know what to do. So, I learned from an early age this is something I was put on this earth for. I didn't share with my parents, but I would act out in different ways. I remember as early as kindergarten attacking the teacher.

During the times of my extreme highs, I believe that is where my addiction formed. Sex, to me, was not a form of showing someone you love them; it was a form of torment. I was tormenting myself as well as others out of control. I write about the life of suffering from this torment in my book "Sexually Driven". Any relationship I entered, I would destroy before they could leave me. I wanted to be loved in my heart, but in my mind, I could not receive that. No one was off limits. Talk about girl code or friend code. I think that is the area I beat myself up the most, thinking I'll never be clean or holy enough deserving of a love of my own and walking the streets at night to 1-900 lines. Just one torment after another. My self-esteem was so low, and I devalued myself. My relationship with people was like a revolving door, and sometimes there were financial transactions.

I didn't even know how to have a relationship in a general atmosphere and surroundings of basic family members. There weren't many hugs, and I love you. You knew you were loved (I guess), but it wasn't shown like "normal" family gatherings. When I am in Hobby Lobby and see signs of the gathering place, it seems so strange to me.

Also, I didn't feel worthy of a healthy and loving of loving relationship. I would push everyone away and would have outbursts. I was throwing dishes, punching walls. Driving dangerously with my partner in the car, threatening to end our lives, and other times attacking with knives. Now this is going to sound crazy, and my trigger was someone trying to show me love. I even had a partner that would go to therapy with me, trying to understand me to be a help to me. However, my outbursts of violence were too much for one to endow. Being promiscuous proceeded as I grew.

One night I was hanging out at the club and met Mr Apple. We spent the night talking and laughing, and nothing out of the ordinary. He offered me a ride home, and I accepted. We pulled over to the side of the road and just talked. Somehow the conversation went to what things we would do that we never did before. Then I asked him, what if I asked him for money? Would he give it to me? He said yes. I asked him for $100, and he gave it to me like it wasn't a problem. That was so interesting and powerful to me at the same time. After hanging out with him, I ran into the house and put the money in the dresser drawer under my clothes. A few days after that, I would look at the money, not believing how easy it was.

I went out to the club again and met Mr Berry, and we sat at the bar all night just talking about different things. Then the conversation subject was sex. I explained I had no desire for sex, which wasn't satisfying. He said he could make me feel excited and could satisfy my needs. I agreed to allow him to try and succeed at this task. We drove to another city and pulled into the parking lot of a motel. It was my first time doing something like this, and I wasn't afraid but a little shame, not wanting anyone to see me there. He went into the front office, came back out, and drove us around to the back where our room was located. He began to perform his acts of sex with me, and as always, there was nothing on my part. I was a basic lay-there type of person that the individual could do whatever they wanted to do. Then I would shower.

He brought me back to the club thinking he showed me, but no, he just made my belief even stronger. There is nothing to sex, and I hate it. I hate myself for allowing someone to touch me.

A lot of times, when I get depressed, I would move furniture around in my place, or I would go for a walk. One day I was walking down the street and ran into Mr Cherry working at a car dealership. He stopped me and struck up a conversation. I invited him over the next day for lunch. I offered to serve him a sandwich or something. He showed up the next day. I made him the sandwich, but we ended up having sex. Of course, he got what he wanted, but I just took my shower and moved on.

Another evening on another walk, I met Mr. Danish. He was a repeat offender. I would hook up with him a few times. One night we were at a public complex; it was late at night, so it didn't matter. The first time I was exploring in the automobile. Then there was a knock on the window by the police. I was so afraid I was going to jail. It made the experience crazier. Then we took it inside.

Interestingly enough, if I did meet someone wanting a real boyfriend/girlfriend relationship, I didn't want to have sex with them. I wanted more. Once I gave myself to someone, I didn't like them anymore. Men are very interesting. They feel they can make you feel all kinds of wonderful. They can have you climaxing over and over. Foreplay and orally, but nothing worked for me. I didn't recognize the pattern right away. I would want to watch porn more and more on my own, and I wanted more self-gratification. I had to self-gratify myself more than once each day, or I truly thought I would die.

I began to look at men as objects to use and didn't have any feelings for them. I was getting high being with the next victim and branching out to females as well. Single or married, spouses of people I knew or partners of people I knew. Bills are paid, flowers are sent to the office, and money is left on the nightstand. It even got to the point where I thought I might star in one of the porn movies or become a prostitute. Just heartless and not caring. One day on one of my walks, I met Mr. Edible. We started talking. He said he was the CEO of a company that was up the street. It was a

24-hour operation, but overnight it was mostly him. One night he called me to come to hang out with him. We talked, and then he started to massage my shoulders and then started caressing my whole body. I just allowed him to explore all areas. Right there in the front lobby, he expressed his feelings that flowed through my flesh. Then I just went to the ladies' room and washed all evidence away as routine as the last and the next.

I learned about phone sex and began calling the 1-900 numbers. Then I became a friend of one of the callers and found out it was a job. I thought, okay, I could do this to make a living because I was on the phone all night anyway. I could make up things to say to keep someone on the line. The trick was you keep them on for a certain amount of time, and then it would cut off so they could call back. Each time they call back, they could be charging more money over and over. I became so detached from reality.

I can give you stories of meeting Mr A to Mr Z, but I think you understand now. The more I hated myself, the more destructive I became. To me, getting AIDS would be a way of my life ending and still going to heaven because I didn't take my life. That's how crazy my thoughts became. I was so disgusted with myself, and I never felt clean. I would shower over and over. To this day, I just don't feel clean enough. I refuse to give myself to anyone. I feel like this is my punishment for never being able to find true love because I don't know how to be intimate with anyone.

Financial Experience:

I learned about payday loans. It's a place you go and apply for a loan, and based on your ability to pay back from your paycheck, they would front you the money. It really isn't based on your ability to pay back because you get into this vicious cycle of being unable to pay. I would get several of them. As soon as they gave me the money, it felt so good. I would automatically think about where I am going to spend the money. There were different people in my life that no matter what, they could help me spend.

These spending binges would satisfy me on a level I can't even explain. However, when payday came, I never would have any money because the payday loan companies collected out of my check before I even got my check. I have lost ownership of cars because they might have been signed over for collateral. I would have to close bank accounts because they had access to them. I have even filed for bankruptcy because I would become over-whelmed. I would tell myself I just needed a fresh start, and everything would be okay.

Unfortunately, if you don't take care of the root of your problems, they will cause a cycle of the same patterns over and over. Yes, that is how my life has been, one horrible cycle.

Chapter Three

Queen and Social Anxiety Disorder

~

Social Anxiety Disorder:

Anxiety is characterized by persistent and exaggerated fear of social situations (such as meeting strangers, dating, or public speaking) in which embarrassment or a negative judgment by others may occur and that causes significant distress, often resulting in an avoidance of such situations and impairment of normal social or occupational activities. I knew I suffered from anxiety in general.

I would go into a panic, my blood pressure would raise to stroke level, and I would have trouble breathing. The ambulance was often called while at work when I had an attack. I think the ladies I work with don't mind because they always talk about how good-looking the firemen are. Yes, they are, lol. I was given meds to calm me down. I didn't relate that to mental illness. However, there was another anxiety I was experiencing.

I just thought I was shy and afraid to be around people in large crowds. I would be assigned to speak in front of a group, and just before it was time for me to come before the people, my heart would start racing, and I would get light-headed, thinking I would faint. My therapist told me I was suffering from a social anxiety disorder. I never knew what that was.

Sometimes the panic attacks would come from a memory of something that seemed like it was happening right then. I was then diagnosed as having Post Traumatic Stress Disorder (PTSD).

Chapter Four

Queen and PTSD

~

Post-traumatic stress disorder: PTSD

A psychological reaction that occurs after experiencing a highly stressful event (such as wartime combat, physical violence, or a natural disaster) outside the range of normal human experience and that is usually characterized by depression, anxiety, flashbacks, recurrent nightmares, and avoidance of reminders of the event.

If you said, PTSD, the first thing that came to my mind is someone that is suffering after being in the military. However, I have learned it is related to having experienced some trauma.

Now I could go out to the clubs and socialize with friends after a few drinks. I felt like a whole different person. However, when sober, I just thought I was shy and afraid to be around others.

My mind was always thinking people really didn't want me around and didn't really like me.

But when there were assignments at work or church or whatever, I would get anxiety that would have my heart racing. It never failed, I'm on the schedule to read a poem or something, and I would just freak out. I remember being part of a prison ministry and being asked to do a read and to share with a group of ladies. When it came to the time I was to speak, my breathing became harder to do. I began to cry, and I became so afraid. My desire is to share with young ladies to encourage them. Maybe it's called public speaking, but it seems like a task that will end my life if I continue pursuing it. Recently, I have been invited to participate in a Toast Master group. It is to help you with public speaking. I have tried it twice before, but I didn't follow through like anything else. Maybe this time, I will.

I also wonder if it was because, as a child, being molested or, as an adult, being manipulated by men in authority. Or the most traumatic thing in my life was the night I went out with my friend to the club, and we were having a good time, and then I ran into Mr Evil. I had been dating someone and met him through that boyfriend. He came into the club and was talking to me and then asked if I would go for a walk with him. I thought nothing of it, and he knew my man. At least he was the man in my mind and heart. So, we went for a walk. Then he said he had to pick up a package for a friend and asked if I would mind coming with him. So, we stopped by his apartment. I was just sitting there, and he went into another room to get the package. He returned to where I was, not with the package but with a gun. He began to ask me different questions about sex, and I did not want to answer. He told me to take my clothes off. I refused and started to struggle with him. I began to yell, and he hit me over and over with the gun. Then he put the gun down, and I thought I could get free, and he had a knife in his hand. He began to rape me, and I thought that night I was going to die. When he finished, he told me I had to come back each week, or he would kill me. I was walking home, and the police drove by. I guess he could see I was all beat up and disoriented. He pulled around, got out, and started asking me if I needed help. I agreed to go with him to the station. I think I was in shock. When we got to the station, they got a female officer and asked me questions and the person's description. I did the best I could, and then one of the officers came back with a picture and asked if it was the person. I freaked out; yes, it was the person.

I had to go to court, and I had to go to counseling. I never completed the counseling. I thought if I just buried it, I would be fine. However, I could be walking uptown just to go shopping, and if I thought I saw that person, my heart would start racing, and I would be so scared. To this day, I have that fear in the back of my mind that I will be found and killed.

Chapter Five

Queen and ADD

~

Attention Deficit Disorder (ADD):

A Developmental disorder that is marked especially by persistent symptoms of inattention (such as distractibility, forgetfulness, or disorganization) or by symptoms of hyperactivity and impulsivity (such as fidgeting, speaking out of turn, or restlessness) or by symptoms of all three and that is not caused by any serious underlying physical or mental disorder.

Now I heard of ADHD, and I thought it was something children suffered from. I didn't know it was something adults suffer from. I would always want to study or start something. There was no problem setting it up. That is just it, and I was always starting. Always setting up. But would never follow through. I'll be honest: I believe the school system pushed me through. I didn't really apply myself. I wish I had done better. I love learning. I love studying the bible. I desire to go back to school to better myself. I feel like I have a second-grader reading level. It is the one thing that shames me. When I'm asked to read aloud if we are in a group, I find out what I will have to read and read it upfront to ensure I know all the words. It is a very exhausting thing to do. I feel like a big liar—an imposter. Also, the other thing is whenever I am in a conversation with someone, and I try so hard to let them get out what they want to say without cutting them off. It never happens, I will cut them off over and over.

Okay, a light bulb just went off. Maybe that is why it's hard to do group settings because I want to cut everyone off in their talking. It isn't easy for real.

No matter how much I try to have some type of order, I just can't focus, and I would just sit and stare into space, wasting away many hours.

I keep experiencing three recurring dreams. I don't know what the connection to dreams is:

- Running and falling off a mountain
- Driving or riding and crashing
- In a house and looking for a secret room

Chapter Six

Queen and Being Saved

~

In my opinion (my opinion and experience alone), I say this next thing. The church wasn't support of someone dealing with mental illness. If you dealt with anything outside of what was considered living the holy life, you were sinning.

At the age of 9 in Arkansas, I received the Holy Spirit. My cousins and I were jumping around, and it hit me for real. They brought me to the car, and I was still under. I tried to live to save but experienced many unsaved life experiences. However, every time I went to church, some preacher called me out for prayer and spoke different things over me. Expressing how anointed and gifted I am. To this day, I have just felt I aborted everything because I didn't understand my part of the responsibility when someone speaks over your life. So, my goal now is to research everything and pray that God makes things clear to me so that I may walk in the plans of the Lord for my life.

Words are spoken over and into my life:

<u>Prophet to the Nations and Seer:</u>

I put these two together, believing they intertwine. I have dreams and see things as if I were watching a movie. The things I see seem to give me a warning. There have been times when I have given others words of encouragement through a dream or thoughts that impressed me.

<u>Intercessor:</u>

Praying on behalf of others. There are times I feel others' pain. I can be around them, and I go into a cry of sadness that I cannot explain. I believe that is mixed with a little discernment as well. Feeling someone else's pain. Because of a lack of knowledge, I was afraid to walk in this area. I thought I had to be perfect to be used. I felt if things were going on with me, I couldn't pray for others, fearing my issue would spill over to them. Maybe that is why the Lord says His people perish for the lack of knowledge, and in all, thy getting gets understanding.

I am hoping the Toast Master's classes that I spoke about in chapter four really help. This way, I will be able to pray in a corporate prayer setting and not fear.

Healing and Encourager:

I put these two together because I believe they intertwine.

Permission to lay hands on others and pray for them. Also, the gift of writing is to encourage others. I feel that is a form of healing emotionally.

As I am creating this book, I know of a pastor who has completed his life coaching course in mental health. That is so encouraging because the more people educate themselves in mental health, the more individuals can get support. Just someone's understanding is priceless! The one thing that is so upsetting is telling someone who deals with depression just to be happy.

I would like to share a poem about how I used to feel. Maybe it is where you or someone you know is at. Be encouraged that things can change for you as well. My daily prayer now is depression is not my portion and the joy of the Lord is my strength. So, I will declare God's word over my life, and if I need it, I will take medication.

∞∞∞

As I sat with a drink in one hand and a bunch of pills in the other,

The plan to end my life didn't work; I'm still here to face another.

Lord, I know I fall short in loving you,

I walk around knowing your word but acting like it's not true.

Help the areas where there is unbelief,

For I realize it is of my privileges that I live beneath.

It's not like I haven't been down this destructive road before

It's like I want to just give up and not be saved anymore

I can't seem to break the strongholds to just give into the flesh,

Instead of praying and waiting on Heaven's best.

Since I have breath in my body, there is still time to turn this thing around.

You will not hear on the news that it is my body they have found.

I will reach out to others to do whatever I can

I realize this is spiritual warfare, and when I've done all I can do, I'll still stand.

I'll make that dinner for two and instead of saving some for tomorrow

I'll take half and go share it with someone who is lonely in their sorrow

Instead of turning on that TV, I'll read your word, and I'll pray

Yes, Lord, I know there is purpose for my life; thank you for another day

∞∞∞

Chapter Seven

Queen Seeking Help

~

On March 3, 2023, I received a text from Walmart that my medication was ready. I still have mixed feelings. I'm ready to get my mind stable, and I know I will feel better. As I shared with the doctor, I know it will make me feel better, but then I start thinking I can do it on my own, and I think about how much it is costing, and I stop taking them. Now that we have a new health plan at work, it really will cost me. Our new insurance does not work in our favor. I heard someone say everything is going up but the paycheck, lol there is some truth in that.

Let me say this. Not everyone needs medication. With me, it helps me to bring my thoughts in and focus and drown out the thoughts that my life will end. It balances the chemicals in my brain. I'm able to have discussions and not be all over the place. One would say, well, that seems like a no-brainer to just be on the meds. That would be easy to say if there wasn't such a stigma to being in therapy and the ignorance of the Christian community.

But then there might be some that ask the question. "If I go on medication, will I be on medication forever?" I have written this book to give my testimony. Not to say, what I share is what will happen for everyone. I share my testimony to give someone hope that they may experience things as I do. I can say no to that for myself. Through therapy and true spiritual guidance, I have learned how to manage my mood swings. I have learned when I am going through stressful moments, I must slow down and give great thought to my surroundings and what is real and what is in my head. I will also say it is important who you surround yourself with. People mean no harm. Sometimes they can alter how you feel. Be around upbeat people. Not someone that will feed depression.

Don't always be alone at home. Get out of the house. Maybe go to a park and take a walk. Sometimes that might be easier said than done. Push, press, and don't give up. I started doing things I was afraid to do. Trust me, and I have a list. I believe one day, I shall be able to do what I believe I am here on earth to do. I will take all that I write about and speak about it before lots of women to encourage them in person. To put a face behind the pen!

I have learned that I must speak up and share what is on my mind. I can get so lost in my thoughts. I used to think I was a realistic person speaking the truth when I, in fact, was a negative person not speaking about life situations. Does medication help me stay levelheaded? Yes. However, having the help of a psychologist and a life coach has helped me work through what my thoughts tell me. One day in the week, I would see the psychiatrist that would follow up with me and monitor my medication. Then another day throughout the week, I would see the psychologist that would follow up, but we would discuss better ways to handle situations. All sessions were not good for me because always I wouldn't say I like answering questions repeatedly, but when I leave the session, I would think back on what was said and end up writing a poem. I truly believe more than ever that God gave me that to help me to de-stress. As well as to encourage others.

Today's doctor's appointment (general wellness check) went a little differently. I had been feeling drained and just not feeling connected to different things going on. Every time I go to the doctor, they give me a form to fill in that has a list of questions regarding my mental status. I never filled it out, but for some reason, I filled it out today. After I met with the doctor, someone from behavioral health came in the room and asked if I wouldn't mind speaking with someone because my numbers were too high on the form I filled out. I said sure. Then we went to another room. As soon as I sat down, I felt myself getting ready to go into that dark place where I withdrew. I said you want me to speak to someone so I don't kill myself when I leave here. To save yourselves. Then the counselor came on. I hate answering questions over and over about how I feel and such things like that. But today was different, and I was able to talk with her. In the end, she asked about introducing me to something else. She spoke with the associate that brought me into the room, stating that there are concerns around death, but it's not suicidal. For the first time, someone listened. Because of my faith, I would not kill myself, but I do have a FEAR of dying. It's overwhelming that I believe I won't be able to prevent it. My anxiety builds, and I think I'm going to die. Or even worse, I will pass out and be buried alive. I had been having dizzy spells as well.

So, the new process they want to try with me is called EMDR (Eye Movement Desensitization Reprocessing). It has something to do with your eye patterns and knowing I still may have negative thoughts, but I will be able to channel the negative thoughts, and I won't get and/or be stuck.

Once I get my finances together and better insurance, I may investigate. Working smarter, not harder, mind frame. If there is a better way of doing things, without such a struggle, of course, why not give it a try?

I would like to share a poem about how I used to feel. Be encouraged again. It's always the darkest before dawn. It will get better. One day at a time. Process is key!

∞∞∞

My desire to live is almost non-existence.

But what can I do about it, for to take my own life would be a sin?

But if depression is a sickness not in my control.

Then maybe God would not hold me responsible and forgive me, and Heaven would still be my home.

I've learned to block my feelings away deep inside

Would it be true to say my life is one big lie?

In all my thoughts, I can't think of one thing good; my past hunts me day and night.

I've even thought maybe a makeover would make things right.

A makeover for the ugliness I wear on the outside and on the in

There's no one to love me; why doesn't God answer that one prayer for all of this to end

People I call my friends sometimes they hurt me, and they don't even know they do

Because I don't tell them because I want to protect them from hurting too

I wasn't a good daughter, mother, nor a good wife

Why, God, why did you give me life?

So many people I know are dying each day.

It seems like I'm being punished I want to go too, and He says no, you must stay.

I don't know my purpose in life; I don't know what's ahead.

I just know each day; I wish I were dead.

I've been abused in so many ways, to tell you; I wouldn't know where to begin.

I wish I could be a virgin again, free from sexual sin.

I wanted to be loved and held, so I believed all the lies the men would say

Girl, you know I love you; I'm never going away.

I can't give you one reason to explain why I feel the way I do, nor to explain why it would justify wanting to die.

I just know there is a pain inside that won't go away nor ease up, and all I can do is cry.

They say if I talk to someone and take the meds, I will be able to see

That there are brighter days ahead for me

Should I really lay it all out there and trust some-one with my deepest thoughts and desires?

Would it really make a difference, or would they just nod their head, pretend to care just because they were hired?

∞∞∞

Chapter Eight

Queen's Passion to Encourage

~

On February 26, 2023, I gave a testimony on how I had been suffering from the torment of suicidal thoughts. After praying, my pastor received a word from the Lord, and I was inspired to write this poem. Maybe you will be encouraged by it. Know that anything the devil comes to you with, he has to get permission. He only has permission to test you and does not have the authority to kill you. Do not give him more power than he has. Through the gift of the Holy Spirit, you have authority. Rebuke fear and anything else that keeps you in bondage and/or torments you. I pray for peace and joy into and over your life!

Queen E. Lacey

∞∞∞∞

You may have permission to test me,

But you don't have authority to kill me.

I shall live and not die;

Devil, you can't torment me anymore because everything you say is a lie.

I shall sleep at night with sweet rest,

Because now I know I have passed the test.

So now I shall walk in the authority given to me,

No longer walking in fear and defeat.

No longer walking in depression with my head hung down,

Devil I serve you notice to get thee behind me now.

I am encouraged even the more

To walk in purpose and declare the works of the Lord.

∞∞∞∞

OTHER WORKS BY THE AUTHOR

IT'S NOT ABOUT RELIGION, GOD WANTS A RELATIONSHIP

Subtitle – God's Love is Unconditional

FROM MY HEART TO YOURS

Subtitle- Nothing Shall Separate You From God's Love

SEARCHING FOR REAL LOVE?

Subtitle – It Won't be Found in Someone Else's Bed

YOUNG HEARTS NEED LOVE TOO

Subtitle – Bringing Awareness to Adults/Parents of Some Struggles of the Youth

FROM THIS DAY FORWARD

Subtitle – Letting the hurts of the past die so you can live in the blessings of today

SEXUALLY DRIVEN

Subtitle – One Church Girl's Struggle with Sexual Addiction and a Desire to Be Loved

SEXUALLY DRIVEN II

Subtitle – Returning to My First Love I

INJURED AND SCARRED BUT NOT BROKEN

Subtitle - Sharing Questions That Lead to My
Wholeness
Workbook

Made in the USA
Columbia, SC
21 November 2023

26840290R10028